I0707271

# 5 Pillars

# Of

# Mental Fitness

## By Dr Peter C. Omoghene

# Legal Notice

5 Pillars of Mental Fitness

Copyright©2020 by Dr Peter Omoghene

# Disclaimer

# Dedication page

This book is dedicated to my lovely wife of 15 years, Mrs. Elo Omoghene and my three wonderful children, Jessica, Peter Jr and Stephanie.

I love you all

Peter C. Omoghene, O.D

# Table of Contents

# Preface

This has always been my passion because much earlier in my practice, I came across several middle-aged patients helpless with mental health issues. At one time, I came across a patient in his early fifties exhibiting early signs of Alzheimer's disease. His wife made me understand that he was a very vibrant soldier who was retired early from the military as a result of this disease. At another time, it was an elderly woman in her mid sixties (accompanied by her daughter) suffering from dementia.

A radiologist friend of mine once told me about an elderly friend of hers living in Tobago who had a wife suffering from Alzheimer's disease and had spent quite a lot of money and time to care for her but the situation still grew worse by the day.

Another very good friend of mine also narrated to me how his own mother suffered from Alzheimer's disease for quite a long while before she finally passed on. The story was very heartbreaking to say the least. I have decided not to disclose any names for privacy reasons.

It breaks my heart to see that so many people are still suffering from what I may classify as preventable illnesses due to lack of knowledge and that is why I have decided to devote my time to write this book, hoping that it will go a long way in preventing such illnesses in many families. Even if it is one life that is saved from reading this book, I have achieved my set objective in writing the book.

The information revealed in this book is not in any way a form of treatment for mental illness but more likely has a strong potential to prevent mental health problems by preserving healthy brain cells and fostering continuous neurogenesis throughout a lifetime.

# Introduction

I believe that the greatest gift a man possesses is his mind and so, it is his responsibility to develop it to its fullest potential. It is important to realize that mental health is equally as important as physical fitness, for a sound mind is one of the most important tools we need to succeed in life. .

We all know the importance of physical fitness and staying healthy throughout our lives, so why do so many people neglect their mental health? What such people fail to realize is that both are connected. Neglecting your mental health can make you less resilient to life's ups and downs, leaving you more likely to make poor lifestyle choices. You can only achieve true success with a sound mind.

Although ageing is inevitable and mental decline is one of the major setbacks of ageing, there are still several things we can do to keep the mind working at peak level and prepare us for our day to day challenges.

The five pillars of mental fitness, developed over the years from scientific research, provides you with all the tools you need to combat age-related mental decline such as Depression, Alzheimer's or Dementia, to mention a few. Using all the information revealed in this book, you are guaranteed of a lifetime of mental fitness.

This book is also very helpful to students as it provides them with all the tools they need to boost their brain power and make studying less stressful. So it is beneficial to everyone that is a lifelong learner.

So what is "the five pillars of mental fitness" all about? It is a comprehensive guide that shows you how to use the 5 pillars to achieve mental fitness throughout life.

Pillar 1 gives you the recommended nutrients needed to build up neurotransmitters and preserve healthy brain cells.

Pillar 2 gives you specific aerobic exercises that ensures sufficient and regular oxygen intake for maximum energy release in the brain.

Pillar 3 provides you with regular mental exercises to keep the brain active so that its cells remain alive preventing age-related and inactivity-related decline. Also if done correctly and regularly, could foster neurogenesis (i.e. formation of new brain cells)

Pillar 4 provides specific lifestyle habits to promote a healthy brain development.

Pillar 5 reveals the heavy metals and toxins that destroy brain cells and deteriorate mental functioning.

I have tried to make all the information in this book as simplified and straight to the point as much as possible so that it could be easy to use.

Dr Peter Omoghene

# CHAPTER I
## Pillar 1

The Five Basic Essential Brain Nutrients:

I choose to start with this because I consider it to be the foundation of the other pillars. Without the right nutrients, the other pillars will not be so effective.

Just as the whole body requires a balanced diet to remain healthy, so does the brain require some basic essential nutrients to remain active and withstand stress.

These essential nutrients can be grouped under five categories;

1) Glucose Balance

11) Essential Fatty acids

111) Phospholipids

1V) Essential Amino Acids

V) Vitamins and minerals

It is advisable to maintain a balance of each of these five nutrients in order to ensure high mental performance.

The brain neurons have to be fed properly with the appropriate nutrients in order to have a rich supply of neurotransmitters for release when necessary.

An under supply of the right nutrients to the neuron can result to poor memory and poor thinking.

Let me give a few examples of neurotransmitters which are derived from nutrients;

Acetylcholine (ACH) is one which is concerned with memory, thinking, motor coordination and sleep. A deficiency or acute lack of acetyl choline (ACH) usually results in memory disorders.

Acetylcholine (ACH) is made from the nutrient choline, which is derived mainly from soybeans, liver, eggs and fish (especially sardines) or from nutritional supplements such as lecithin, phosphotidyl choline or choline itself, vitamin B5 is also essential for the formation of Acetylcholine (ACH).

Some other neurotransmitters derived from nutrients are: serotonin which is derived from tryptophan, an amino acid found in turkey, chicken and milk.

Epinephrine is derived from tyrosine found in most food. Dopamine and Nor epinephrine (which are also key brain stimulant) are produced from tyrosine. Other neurotransmitters derived from nutrients include nitric oxide and gamma-ammine butyric acid.

Before we continue, it is very important to note that although exercising the brain (mental exercise) helps develop and build it to grow bigger, it's maximum growth and development cannot be achieved without the use of the essential nourishments mentioned above. It can be compared to muscle building which has a limited development without the use of essential proteins (Amino acids to be precise). You will discover that when super supplements are added to a largely natural food diet, there is a remarkable improvement in mental ability and achievement.

Glucose Balance

Keeping your blood sugar balance is probably the most important factor in maintaining an even energy, mood and concentration as well as many other factors. Glucose is the brain's favorite food.

When an individual is stimulated mentally or physically there is usually an increased blood flow to billions of brain and body cells.

This results in an increased rate at which oxygen combines with food substances especially glucose to release energy in the brain and body cells.

In other words, the 'burning' of glucose (the brain's major fuel) results in the release of energy for increased mental activity.

However, with limited oxygen or glucose in the brain, this very vital process slows down, so there is therefore less energy for mental activity and resultantly your thinking and memory is not as efficient as it is supposed to be. Occasionally, when this occurs, some people misinterpret it as Alzheimer's disease or senile dementia (when present in the elderly).

Your brain is fueled each hour with about a teaspoon of glucose. For this reason, when the glucose level in the blood drops below normal, an individual is likely to experience a whole host of symptoms including mental (physical) fatigue, poor concentration, irritability, nervousness, depression, excessive sweating, thirst, headaches and digestive problems.

Very important note; Glucose deprivation injures cells in the hippocampus, a brain area devoted to memory and mood control. Under stress conditions, most of the glucose is diverted from the brain to other vital body organs and the muscles causing severe harm to brain function.

Sustained stress resulting in glucose deprivation in the brain can lead to brain cell starvation and resultantly an unreliable memory and poor thinking.

Controlling blood sugar levels:

In controlling your blood sugar levels, it is advisable to eat foods with to moderate glycemic index.

Glycemic index is the scientific measurement of how the insulin (from the pancreatic gland) responds to the intake of a particular food.

The insulin helps to regulate the sugar in the blood, keeping it normal.

Foods classified under low glycemic index usually trigger a low insulin response while that with high glycemic index evoke a high insulin response.

Low glycemic index foods include fish, meat, green vegetables, peanuts, soybeans, eggs, milk, beans, fruit sugar (pure factor) peas, and yogurt)

Moderate glycemic index foods include sweet potatoes, oranges pineapple juice, nuts, whole grain bread, grapes, brown rice, bran cereal.

High glycemic index foods include carrots, corn flakes, white bread, millet, white rice, refined flower pasta cakes, bananas, candy, cookies (and other pastries).

Note; Foods with low glycemic index can form part of our regular diet especially when taken with nutritional supplements {multivitamins and multiminerals}.

Foods with moderate glycemic index should not be taken regularly. High glycemic index foods should be seriously controlled and eaten once in a while.

Finally it is also advisable to prevent low blood sugar by eating several small meals a day this will also ensure easy digestion and absorption of such food substances by the body.

Note; It is highly advisable to give the brain its quota of glucose and oxygen to make it much more efficient to handle mental tasks

Essential Fatty Acids

Fatty acids are referred to as essential because they are not produced in the body and they are very vital for the smooth functioning of the brain and nervous system.

The balance of fats is very critical to the brains structure and function. So for brain health, both omega 3 and omega 6 fats must be present in your diet.

Omega 3 fats contain docosahexanoic acids (DHA) and flex oil contains eicosapentanoic acids (EPA).

These are two very important fatty acids, which are of immense value for a healthy brain functioning.

Polyunsaturated oils provide the 2 essential fats omega 3 and omega 6.

Omega 3 fats

The best sources of Omega 3 fats are fish (especially the more oily fish such as mackerel, herring and salmon) and flax seeds (also known as linseeds) and their oils. Also, it can be derived from linolenic acid.

Note; The level of the omega 3 fats (DHA and EPA) both found in fish oils are markers for intelligence.

Studies have shown that the blood levels of these essential fats correlate with intellectual performance and learning ability at the age of five.

The world health organization now recommended that baby formula feeds include these oils. Flaxseed and chia are the best sources of omega 3. The best seeds oil for omega 3 fats is hemp, pumpkins, evening primrose oil, flax seeds, chia seeds.

It is important to note that carnivorous fish and their oils also contain Eicosapentanoic Acid (EPA) and Docosahexanoic Acid (DHA). Eating too much saturated fat also promotes the production of less desirable prostaglandins called pg E2, which are involved in inflammatory and clotting mechanisms in the body.

The prostaglandins derived from omega 3 fats are essential for proper brain function. They also promote good vision, learning ability, coordination and mood as well as countless other body functions.

For an improved memory, omega 3 fats in supplementation forms such as fish oil capsules is advisable, usually, a daily dose of 400 mg to 500 mg of EPA and DHA produce highly desirable results after several weeks.

These are also essential for mental health. Of all the body tissues, the brain has the highest proportion of omega 6 fats. They are part of nervous tissues and influence brain functions. Also adding evening primrose oil to the diet dramatically in the long term improves memory (this is because these oils are precursors of and every other major body functions.  They are also a part of cell membranes.

Due to its reported effects on memory, evening primrose oil was given to Alzheimer's patients in a controlled trial. Once again, highly significant improvements in memory and mental functions were registered.

 This family of fat comes exclusively from seeds and their oils.  The best seed oils are hemp, pumpkin, sunflower, safflower, walnut, soybean and soy, wheat germ oil, corn oil. Omega 6 series is always found in linoleic acid.

It is also noteworthy that evening primrose capsules (500 mg) daily protect against arterial blockage, heart attack and stroke;


Phospholipids (Memory Molecules)

These are phosphorous containing fats which although can be produced in the body, can also be derived directly from the diet. This substance is essential for healthy cell membranes throughout the body and brain. It also helps cell membranes stay flexible for the easy entry of oxygen and nutrients and the exit of wastes. Almost 60 percent of our brain is fat, which is desperately needed to produce and transmit electrical energy.

(i) Phosphatidyl Serine (PS)

This is a vital part of the structure of the brain receptor site, which is easy to take as a nutritional supplement. PS which is also known as memory molecule has a genuine boost to the brainpower. It improves dramatically the memory, learning ability, concentration and thinking power.

The body usually makes sufficient phosphatidyl serine until middle age or beyond when production slows down. This affects thinking and remembering.

However, during periods when the body production of PS has slowed down, it can be derived directly by eating organ meats (about 50mg in a day), also from nutritional supplements. PS supplements help new cell membrane flexibility and flushes away accumulated wastes. It can be characterized as a biological brain detergent that creates more receptors on brain cells – upgrading communication between nerve cells, corrects stress – related nerve damage and recharges the ability to think and remember.

Research has shown that PS apparently reverses roughly twelve years of mental decline.

PS can be derived from soy lecithin but it is impossible to derive enough PS by ingesting soy lecithin. So to get enough PS, it is advisable to derive it from individual nutrients in the body such as the sulfur containing amino acids, methionine essential fatty acids, folic acids (from green vegetables and other plant issues) and vitamin B-12 (from live kidney, beef).

Foods richest in methionine are eggs, fish, liver, milk, whole grains, corn, nuts, rice and seeds (it is also advisable to reduce alcohol consumption to the barest minimum, as alcohol destroys methionine

Daily Requirement

 Usually it is advisable to take 100mg of PS, three times daily as a regular part of your diet.

An inexpensive way of deriving PS from the source ingredients is by eating fresh fish three times a week, along with fresh vegetables.

(ii) Choline and Dimethyl amino ethanol (DMAE)

The key brain chemical for memory is acetyl choline (ACH), a neurotransmitter that is derived from nutrient choline

DMAE – is a source of choline that is storable in infinitesimal amounts in brain neurons. It tends to disappear as we age.

ACH is a partly responsible for how we connect sensory information with memories and then appropriately. However you don't make acetyl choline (ACH) by eating choline. Vitamins B5 is essential for the formation of acetylcholine (ACH) in the body.

Major sources of choline include eggs, fish (especially sardines). Other sources includes liver, soybeans, peanuts and nuts,

It is also important to note that phosphatidyl choline (PC) which you get from eggs and lecithin is the most suitable form of this vital brain nutrient (Side benefit: Choline improves liver function)

Since lecithin (Key ingredient is choline) or PC is an emulsifier that breaks down fats, it helps in coping with fat deposits in the blood vessels.

DMAE.

Function:

(i) It improves attention span, learning ability, ability to remember stored facts, and boosts overall intelligence.

(ii) It even promotes a quicker and better sleep.

Sources:

Sardines and anchovies are the richest sources of DMAE. DMAE supplements are however available.

Theory on how DMAE works:

(i) It speeds up the brain's synthesis and turnover of a key neurotransmitter acetylcholine, essential for thinking and memory.

(ii) It blocks the metabolism of choline in body tissues, increasing the amount of this nutrient entering the brain and stimulating brain cell receptors.

By these 2 actions, it speeds up mental processes.

Acetyl–L–carnitine

This is another brain enhancer that is very useful in improving the mental performance of young and healthy people as well as that of the middle agers and above, who are losing their ability to synthesize this nutrient.

It energizes the brain, slows down its aging and protects brain cells from free radical damage.

Action

It increases our natural capacity to transport fat across cell membranes so that the energy furnaces each cell or mitochondria, have more fuel to burn. Acetyl-L-Carnitine carries out the same functions as plain carnitine, the body's own substance, but does them even better.

Daily Requirement:

Research experiments have shown that by taking 1,500mg of Acetyl –L–carnitine daily for a prolonged period of time (about 12 weeks and above ) produces a very remarkable improvement in thinking ability, memory and a relaxed state of mind.

The benefits derived from Acetyl–L–carnitine always persist long after supplementation stops.

Essential Amino Acid

These are the building blocks of protein. We have 8 "essential Amino Acids''. The better the balance of amino acids expressed as unit net protein usability (USP), the more you can make use of such proteins.

A few ways can also be used to increase protein content. For instance, combining legumes with rice.

It is also noteworthy that a man needs to eat 3-4 servings of high protein content foods every day, while a woman needs to eat only 2-3 servings a day.

A typical day allotment of protein for a man might therefore include an egg for breakfast (10g), a 200g salesman steak for lunch (40g), and a serving of beans with dinner (20g) other good senses of protein ( especially for vegetarians ) include "seed" food such as nuts, beans, lentils, peas, maize or the germ of grains such as wheat or oat. Also, flower food such as broccoli.

Protein Supplementation

High quality protein occasionally taken for breakfast help supercharge the mental energy before noon.

Also, a light dinner with foods rich in the amino acid tyrosine can raise blood sugar level and improve rapidly the quality of your thinking (for non- diabetics)

Note: Tyrosine-rich foods include cottage cheese, turkey, wheat germ, tuna fish and duck meat.

Note:

Tyrosine is important because it helps produce key brain stimulants nor epinephrine and dopamine

Glutamic Acid (Brain fuel):

This is an amino acid, one of two forms of "fuel" that the brain uses for developing needed energy.

Research has shown that glutamic acid, when taken by children in large amounts (because it has difficulty crossing the blood–brain barrier of about 12 g daily with food over a prolonged period of time of about 6months  to a year improves thinking ability (problem solving  ability)

Requirement

For adults, a daily dose of 1000mg to 4,000mg of amino acid L-Glutamine usually produces a remarkable result.

The natural substance, L–Glutamine is available in tablet or capsule forms.

Several studies have shown that a high protein breakfast is very valuable in keeping the individual mentally alert until noon.

A high level protein includes fortified milk and eggs.

It is important to note that tryptophan, an essential amino acid (one your body can't make) is difficult to absorb into the brain. It is found in turkey milk peanuts, Pumpkins and sesame seeds.

However, with a high carbohydrate meal, tryptophan has less competition from other amino acids and so gets through.

Protein and sleep

Studies have shown that the amount of tryptophan in the brain and blood plasma determines the amount of serotonin, a neuro transmitter in the brain. Serotonin induces sleepiness and reduces sensitivity to pain.

Protein and Stress

Incessant stress causes life supporting protein to be drawn out from the various organs and tissues where they are stored to be used up.

In other words, for highly stressed individuals, an extra supply of protein is needed to meet the body and brain's inordinate demand for it.

Vitamins and Minerals (Intelligent Nutrients)

Vitamins and minerals (trace elements) are very important nutrients, which are required by (the body) brain in minute quantities at a time and aid in the many physiological processes within the (human body) brain.

It is very important to note that the deficiency of one or several of these essential nutrients can affect your thinking efficiency and memory drastically. Vitamin–rich foods such as whole meat products, fresh fruit and vegetables, meat and fish, milk and soy products, nuts and fresh herbs contain everything needed by the human body.

The proper supply of vitamins and minerals however is often not guaranteed these days through imbalanced food intake due to incorrect diet, severe stress at work or in the home, high physical stress or dieting.

Fundamentally, it can be said that the more stressful the environment, the more difficult it is to obtain the proper supply of vitamins and minerals.

For this reason, it is very necessary to obtain a balanced mixture of vitamins from dietary supplements.

The intellectual (and physical) development of children could be predicated with a high degree of accuracy on the basis of their nutritional status during the pre-school years.

Every one of the fifty known essential nutrients with the exception of vitamins D has a role to play in promoting brain function.

In highly stressed individuals, an extra supply of vitamin A is essential for recovery to normal.

The B–complex group of vitamins is one of the most vital groups of vitamins for mental health.

Reason: The B-vitamins ensure an efficient transportation of oxygen inside the brain and body cells.

Deficiency of one of the eight B–vitamins will rapidly affect how you think and feel.

Reason: This is because the brain uses a large amount of these nutrients.

Important Note: The B-Vitamins are water soluble and rapidly pass out of the body so we need a regular intake throughout the day.

An excellent source of vitamin B-complex includes a combination of brewer's yeast and desiccated liver.

B-vitamins combine with choline to increase the production of acetyl choline (ACH) neurotransmitters in the brain.

Important Note: Without B-complex, carbohydrates & foods cannot be utilized to produce useful energy for the nerve cells.

Vitamin B-1 (Thiamin)

This helps to upgrade the memory by several of its roles in the brain. It controls translating glucose into energy in the brain and nervous system.

Thiamin helps to synthesize fatty acids (a very essential brain nutrient) in the nerve cells. It also helps to synthesize acetyl choline (ACH) (a very important neurotransmitter) in the brain.

Important Note; Vitamin B-1 (Thiamine) becomes more effective in memory enhancement when taken with choline.

Choline, the precursor to the neurotransmitter acetylcholine is derived mainly from lecithin, which is, in turn derived from soy or egg yolks (other sources are wheat germ, brewer's yeast, peanuts and meat.

Sufficient intake of vitamin B-1 ensures that many other brain foods are digested and absorbed.

Thiamin is also part of the various enzymes which aid carbohydrate metabolism. About 2 mg of vitamin B-1 taken daily for some week can produce a remarkable important in brain activity.

The best sources of vitamin B-1 are mackerel, salmon, egg yolk, liver and walnuts.

Vitamin B-1 (Thiamin) supplementation Research has shown that taking low potency vitamin B-1 tablet with meal for a short period of time such as between 6 days to 9 days can be very helpful for efficient brain activity.

Note; However, it is best to take individual B-vitamin fractions (Such as vitamin B-1) with the entire vitamin B-complex)

Daily Requirement: 2 mg of vitamin B-1 daily is very useful

Vitamin B-3 (Niacin)

Vitamin B-3 has a tremendous influence on memory and thinking ability. It does this by dilating the brain arteries and capillaries thereby allowing greater entry of oxygen-carrying blood.

However, it is advisable to take niacin with a B- complex supplement containing between 50–100mg of the major B-family members.

In addition to widening arteries, niacin help to enhance brain function by being an important part of a co-enzyme called NAD which helps to energize the brain.

An insufficient supply of niacin makes NAD incomplete so there is a slow down on the metabolic reaction and interrupts the energy supply for the brain cells.

It is important to note that side effect of niacin includes flush, itching or prickly skin for a few minutes.

Also, sustained release of niacin causes some liver damage. So it has to be used with some measure of caution, preferably under the supervision of a knowledgeable health professional.

As said before, It is important to combine niacin intake with the major B-complex family in order to increase the rate of brain metabolism (i.e. the rate at which the brain makes use of oxygen and nutrients.)

Vitamin B-5 (Pantothenic acid): Vitamin B-5 combines with choline to increase the formation of neurotransmitter acetyl chorine (Ach) (useful for enhancing memory).

It helps in processes that release energy in the brain for increased mental activity.

The best food and supplement sources of vitamin B-5 are royal jelly, whole brown rice, corn, egg yolk, peas, sunflower seeds, lentils, eggs, bee pollen, wheat germ and whole wheat.

Pantothenic acid is necessary as an enzyme component to synthesize fatty acids and in metabolism of fat, carbohydrates and amino acids which are very vital to increase brain activity.

Vitamin B6 (Pyridoxine): Pyridoxine is important in brain function as it is essential for the manufacture of neurotransmitters.

It is also necessary for the conversion of amino acids into serotonin and takes part in the formation of hemoglobin.

A deficiency in this important neurotransmitter can cause depression and other problems.

Reason: This is because a deficiency of vitamin B6 and Zinc cause dendrites to shrivel and die.

Vitamin B12 (Cyanocobalamin)

This vitamin helps in protein and fat metabolism.

Note: Of all the B-vitamins, this best known for enhancing memory. It is very important for the health of the nerve cells so it accelerates the rate of learning.

Deficiency of vitamin B-12 can invite an array of mental and emotional problems such a memory loss, difficulty in thinking, hallucination depression and confusion.

The best dietary sources of vitamin B12 are eggs, legumes, organ meat, cheese, liver, fish and shell fish.

However, vitamin B12 is sufficient to get absorbed by the body unless the stomach secretes enough "intrinsic factor" to make the process easier.

It is noteworthy that the richest sources of vitamin B–12 are liver kidney, fish, eggs and beef (Salmon, mackerel, sardines, and herring.)

At this point, it is very important to note that fish is very important for the health of the brain.

The best sources of vitamin B12 include royal jelly, peanuts wheat germ, brewer's yeast, desiccated liver.

Daily Requirement: It is advisable to take between 50mg to 100mg of vitamin B- complex daily on a regular basis.

Note: Fish is regarded as one of the most important brain food – as it contains almost all the nutrients essential for healthy brain activity. It contains vitamin B12, B-1, phospholipids (Choline, DMAE), methionine, Iron (Called heme) and essential fatty acids (Omega 3 fats; DHA & EPA).

Vitamins C and E (Antioxidants)

Your brain and nervous system are made up of protein, phospholipids and essential fats, all of which can be damaged by oxidants (the body's own nuclear waste).

The brain being more than half-fat becomes easily oxidized.

Sources of oxidants: The three factors which introduce these oxidants into the body are fried food, smoking and pollution.

These oxidants now cause a chain reaction of damage to the essential fats attached to the phospholipids in the nerve cell membranes.

Free radicals are bi-products of normal oxygen metabolism in the body and these wreck havoc on other cells resulting in disease and aging.

Anti-oxidants help absorb free radicals protecting us from the harm they cause.

We have several anti-oxidants but the most popular are vitamins A, C and E

There is no organ or area of the body that contains more unsaturated fats than the CNS. This makes the CNS a prime target for attack by free radicals. So vitamin C which is powerful antioxidants serves as a free radical fighter in the CNS.

The human body has a natural pump which draws vitamin C out of the blood circulation and highly concentrates it in the spinal fluid.

A second pump draws vitamin C out of the spinal cord and concentrates it to surround and bathe the spinal cord, nerves cells and the brain with a total concentration much greater than in all other body fluids. Several researches have shown that vitamin C can indeed boost an individual's mental performance.

Without any doubt, vitamin C ensures a better brain health and thinking ability.

Additional function of vitamin C: It is also very important to note that apart from ensuring a better brain health, vitamin C, if taken several times daily and consistently for a prolonged period of time help to strength the walls of the blood vessels thereby correcting any signs of arteriosclerosis.

This eventually ensures that there is a powerful blood flow reaching all areas of the body and brain.

Daily Requirement: It is advisable to take at least 500 mg of vitamin C after each meal and if possible three times daily.

Very good sources of vitamin C are orange or mango juice and fresh fruits generally.

Important Note: Vitamin E which is also a very powerful antioxidant helps to process unsaturated fatty acids important to brain health and activity.

The presence of any cardiovascular disease will definitely result in hardening and blockage in arteries, which supply key nutrients to the brain.

 In conditions like these, the absence of a good supply of antioxidants such as vitamin C and E will result in the brain cells being completely damaged by free radicals.

Sources of Vitamins C and E: Vitamin E is abundant in wheat germ, seeds, nuts, fish and beans. Vitamin C is abundant in fresh fruits, tomatoes, berries and peppers.

Researchers have also shown that higher percentage of anti-oxidants in the blood is associated with better memory performance.

Vitamin E is the most important of the fat based anti-oxidants since it prevents chain reactions of damage caused when oxidants enter the brain.

Minerals and Trace Elements

These are required by the body and brain in minute quantities.

The brain functions depend on adequate intake of magnesium, calcium, zinc and a few other essential minerals.

Boron: Boron helps improve thinking ability and remembering by improving our alertness and concentration.

Research has shown that a deficiency in Boron results in a decline in alertness and concentration which resultantly affects the memory.

Source: Boron can be found in fruits and vegetables.

Requirement: A daily consumption of 3mg of boron for a prolonged period of time also enhances memory.

Deficiency: Boron deficiency affects motor performance i.e. there is usually a slow reaction time to a stimulus

Zinc: Zinc and iron also cause an impressive improvement in memory. Action of Zinc: Zinc helps to activate at least 80 nervous system enzymes involved in the thinking process. So it is very essential for effective thinking,

Zinc is also required to digest and utilize protein (from which the body issue is made).

Research showed that the blood level of zinc is less in senile individuals than much younger individuals. So it is advisable that the intake of zinc be more regular in senile individuals to help boost their thinking ability.

Zinc and copper compete for the same absorption sites in the intestine. So excessive amounts of zinc can knock out the absorption of copper.

A reasonable ratio for copper to zinc intake should is 2mg to 30mg

The deficiency of zinc and vitamin B6 can also cause dendrites to shrivel and die.

The deficiency of copper and vitamin B6 can also cause weakness in mental performance.

Requirement

Daily intake of between 25mg to 30mg of zinc (Usually in the form of tablets) for a prolonged period of time can produce a remarkable mental efficiency.

Sources of Zinc: Red meat, egg yolk, oats, fish, beans, wheat germ, sunflower seeds.

Iron (memory mineral): Just like zinc, iron supplements cause an impressive improvement in memory.

Research studies have revealed the importance of increasing the intake of these minerals.

One mineral or trace element can upset the ratios of minerals to one another, so it is advisable to take them at separate times and usually under the guidance of a knowledgeable health professional.

It is very important to note that taking iron together with zinc as supplements daily will not produce a significant improvement in memory as iron and zinc interfere with each other's absorption. However, they don't when they are part of the entire diet.

Requirement: A daily intake of 30mg of iron supplement can improve the memory remarkably.

However, separating the intake of iron supplement at one time and the intake of zinc supplement at another time will produce the desired result. In order words, it is advisable that one of the mineral supplements be taken in the morning with breakfast while the other is taken in the evening with dinner.

Sources of iron: Red meat, chicken, beans, fish, oats, wheat germ, sunflower seeds, egg yolk.

Action of Iron: Each molecule of hemoglobin (iron–rich protein in the red blood cells) contains about four atoms of iron that make oxygen carrying possible.

If there are two few red blood cells or they are too small, they can't deliver enough oxygen to every cell in the body especially the brain which requires much oxygen for efficient mental activity.

Also, the low quality of the hemoglobin can be equally limiting.

So enough iron is required for the formation of quality hemoglobin in the red blood cells in order to improve their oxygen carrying capacity especially to blood cells where they are needed most such as the brain cells during high mental activity.

Iron's major task involves facilitating the blood's hemoglobin to carry oxygen to the cells and helping the body's protein to function properly.

Very Important note: Any surplus iron just remains unabsorbed in the blood stream and even constitute a risk in the sense that when oxidized it is converted to free radicals which attack healthy cells.

In other words, excess iron in the bloodstream is dangerous.

So, unlike zinc supplementation, iron supplementation must be taken under the supervision of a knowledgeable health professional.

In fact, it is likely that deficiency in vitamin B12 will result in poor thinking ability and memory than iron deficiency.

Iron supplements are only advisable after medical test has been conducted on the individual and an iron deficiency established.

Reason:  Excess iron in the blood stream will eventually lead to liver cirrhosis (i.e. liver injury and degeneration).

Improving Iron absorbability: Research has shown that daily intake of between 200mg to 500mg of vitamin C can increase iron absorbability. The kind of iron found in fish and meat is about 40% absorbed.  Rich sources of Iron: fish, meat, chicken and liver

Calcium and Magnesium: A combination of calcium and magnesium play an essential role in the nervous system.

When you combine 600 mg of calcium and 400 mg of magnesium, they help slowly put you to sleep.

Magnesium forms part of a number of enzymes that aid protein, fat and carbohydrate metabolism.

# CHAPTER 2
## Pillar 2

Specific Aerobic Exercises

What is aerobic exercise?

Aerobic exercise is any form of physical exercise involving the regular or rhythmic movements of the arms or legs or both that leads to improved oxygen intake into the lungs for onward transmission to the brain and several other vital organs of the body.

It should be noted at this point in time that two-thirds of the oxygen inhaled is utilized by the brain, while the remaining one-third is utilized by the other organs of the body.

Aerobic exercise improves the blood circulation throughout the entire body thereby ensuring that oxygen and other vital nutrients get to every organ in the body.

Research has shown that regular aerobic exercises boost memory. A year of moderate exercise doesn't just strengthen the muscles — it also fortifies the brain. A memory center in the brain called the hippocampus shrinks a little bit each year with age, but older adults who walked routinely for a year actually gained hippocampus volume, researchers report in a study.

Study participants who got their heart rates up performed slightly better on a memory test and had higher levels of a brain-aiding molecule called BDNF, the researchers found.

How does it do this?

It does this by aiding the production of nor epinephrine, a neurotransmitter used by the brain to transfer short term memory into neocortex for long term storage.

It stimulates the synthesis of the hormone called "nerve growth factor" needed to repair neurons.

A brain that is deprived of regular supply of oxygen cannot perform as efficiently as one with consistent and regular supply.

Benefits of Aerobic Exercise

In addition to increasing mental clarity, aerobic exercises reduces risk of  obesity, heart disease, high blood pressure, type 2 diabetes (helps to control blood sugar levels) , stroke and certain types of cancer.

Although the full benefits of aerobic exercise is not as received under these conditions:

(1) When it is done less than 30minutes in a day: It is important that your exercise does not go less than 30minutes in a day, even if you have to break it down into 3 10minute workouts.

(2) When it is not regular: In order for aerobic exercise to be effective, it has to be regular. The secret to a successful regular aerobic workout is to make it as exciting and as much fun as possible. That way, you can always look forward to it and keep it up.

(3) When it becomes longer than 2hours at a time: The aim of the workout in the first place becomes defeated. The important body fuel, glucose becomes exhausted resulting to fatigue of the muscles.

 You can start out as slow as necessary and work your way up to at least 30 minutes of moderate exercise a day. And no need to worry, those 30 minutes a day can even be broken up into 3 10-minute workouts a day. Some ideas for squeezing in extra physical activity include taking the stairs at work, parking as far away from buildings as you can to walk more, and working in your yard or garden.

When you do so, you are assured of an enhanced mental performance.


Aerobic exercises and cardiac patients

For cardiac patients, aerobic exercise is also very useful as long as it is done properly in the right amount and at the right time after a careful cardiac evaluation.

It is important to note that regular aerobic exercises improve cardiovascular fitness; it reduces the cardiac rate at rest so that the heart works less strenuously and more efficiently.

Important Note

If an individual has any type of heart problem, it is advisable that he consults a cardiologist to determine if exercise is safe for him, and if so what type and also what should be the extent of the exercise.

Exercise is not advisable for an individual who has severe heart failure and is short of breath at rest, or suffers from certain cardiac rhythm disturbances, or experience angina at rest or at night, or who has aortic stenosis (a valvular disorder)

Some exercises that are particularly good for cardiac patients are dancing, biking and walking.

Exercises that are particularly bad for such patients are isometric ones, particularly those involving the use of the arms such as lifting of weights, shoveling, and sawing wood.

Recommended duration for aerobic exercise:

How long should the average adult exercise every day?

For most healthy adults, the Department of Health and Human Services recommends these exercise guidelines:

Aerobic activity: Get at least 150 minutes a week of moderate aerobic activity or 75 minutes a week of vigorous aerobic activity. You also can do a combination of moderate and vigorous activity. The guidelines suggest that you spread out this exercise during the course of a week.

Strength training: Do strength training exercises at least twice a week. No specific amount of time for each strength training session is included in the guidelines.

Moderate aerobic exercise includes such activities as speed walking, swimming and mowing the lawn. Vigorous aerobic exercise includes such activities as running and aerobic dancing. Strength training can include use of weight machines, or activities such as rock climbing or farming activities.

As a general goal, aim for at least 30 minutes of physical activity every day. If you want to lose weight or meet specific fitness goals, you may need to exercise more. Want to aim even higher? You can achieve more health benefits if you ramp up your exercise to 290 minutes a week.

Short on long periods of time? Even brief periods of activity offer benefits. For instance, if you can't fit in one 30-minute walk, try three 10-minute walks instead. What's most important is making regular physical activity part of your lifestyle.

Recommended frequency of aerobic exercise:

Aerobic exercise: What's the best frequency for workouts?

Which is better — 30 minutes of aerobic exercise every day, or one hour of aerobic exercise three times a week?

Answer:

Longer, less frequent sessions of aerobic exercise have no clear advantage over shorter, more frequent sessions of activity. Any type of aerobic activity contributes to cardiovascular fitness. In fact, even divided "doses" of activity — such as three 11-minute walks spread throughout the day — offer aerobic benefits. What's most important is making regular physical activity part of your lifestyle.

For most healthy adults, the Department of Health and Human Services recommends:

At least 150 minutes a week of moderate aerobic activity (think brisk walking or swimming) or 75 minutes a week of vigorous aerobic activity (such as running) — preferably spread throughout the week. Activity sessions should be at least 10 minutes long.

Strength training exercises at least twice a week.

If you want to lose weight or meet specific fitness goals, you may need to increase your activity even more.

The bottom line is the more active you are in general, the greater the benefits — whether you choose longer, less frequent workouts or shorter, more frequent workouts.

Recommended intensity of aerobic exercise:

Get the most from your workouts by knowing how to determine your exercise intensity:

When you exercise, are you working hard or hardly working? Working out at the approved intensity can assist you can get the most out of your physical activity — making sure you're not overdoing or even under doing it. Here's a look at what exercise intensity means and how to make it work for you.

Understanding exercise intensity

When you engage in aerobic activity, such as walking or biking, exercise intensity correlates with how difficult the activity feels to you. Exercise intensity also is reflected in how rapid your heart is working.

There are two basic ways to measure exercise intensity:

How you feel. Exercise intensity is a subjective measure of how tough physical activity feels to you while you're doing it — your perceived exertion. Your perceived level of exertion may be different from what someone else feels doing the same exercise. For example, what feels to you like a difficult run can feel like an easy workout to someone who's more physically fit.

Your heart rate: Your heart rate offers a more objective look at exercise intensity. In general, the higher your heart rate during physical activity, the higher the exercise intensity.

Studies show that your perceived exertion correlates well with your heart rate. So if you think you're working hard, your heart rate is likely elevated.

You can use either way for determining exercise intensity. If you like technology, a heart rate monitor might be a useful device for you. If you feel you're in tune with your body and your level of exertion, you likely will do well without a monitor.

Choosing your exercise intensity:

How do you know how hard you should be exercising? For most healthy adults, the Department of Health and Human Services recommends these exercise guidelines:

Aerobic activity: Get at least 150 minutes a week of moderate aerobic activity — such as brisk walking, swimming or mowing the lawn — or 75 minutes a week of vigorous aerobic activity — such as running or aerobic dancing. You can also do a combination of moderate and vigorous activity, preferably spread throughout the course of a week.

Strength training: Do strength training exercises at least twice a week. Consider free weights, weight machines or activities that use your own body weight — such as rock climbing or heavy gardening. The amount of time for each session is up to you.

So think about your reasons for exercising. Do you want to improve your fitness, lose weight, train for a competition, or a combination of these? Your answer will help determine the appropriate level of exercise intensity.

To reap the most health benefits from exercise, your exercise intensity must generally be at a moderate or vigorous level. For weight loss, the more intense your exercise, or the longer you exercise, the more calories you burn. However, balance is important. Overdoing it can increase your risk of soreness, injury and burnout. If you're new to regular exercise and physical activity, you may need to start out at a light intensity and gradually build up to a moderate or vigorous intensity.

How to determine your exercise intensity by how you feel

Simple ways to help you out:

Light exercise intensity

Light activity feels easy. Here are signs that your exercise intensity is at a light level:

You have no noticeable changes in your breathing pattern.

You don't break a sweat (unless it's very hot or humid).

You can easily carry on a full conversation or even sing.

Moderate exercise intensity

Moderate activity feels more difficult. Here are signs that your exercise intensity is at a moderate level:

Your breathing is more rapid, but you're not out of breath.

You feel a light sweat after about 10 minutes of activity.

You can carry on a conversation, but you can't sing.

Vigorous exercise intensity

Vigorous activity feels challenging. Here are clues that your exercise intensity is at a vigorous level:

Your breathing is deep and rapid.

You develop a sweat after a few minutes of activity.

You can't say more than a few words without pausing for breath.

Overexerting yourself

Beware of pushing yourself too hard too often. If you're short of breath, in pain or can't work out as long as you'd planned, your exercise intensity is probably higher than your fitness level allows. Slow down a bit and build intensity gradually.


Aerobic Interval Training:

Interval training is a powerful tool for novice exercisers and accomplished athletes alike. Here's how it works:

What is interval training?

Interval training is simply alternating periods of intense activity with intervals of lighter activity.

Take walking. If you're in good shape, you might incorporate short periods of jogging into your regular fast walks. If you're less fit, you might alternate leisurely walking with periods of faster walking. For example, if you're walking outdoors, you could walk faster between certain landmarks.

What can interval training do for me?

Whether you're a beginner exerciser or you've been exercising for years, interval training can help you improve your workout routine. Consider the benefits:

You'll burn more calories. The more vigorously you exercise the more calories you'll burn— even if you increase intensity for just a few minutes at a time.

You'll improve your exercise intensity. As your cardiovascular fitness improves, you'll be able to exercise longer or with more intensity. Imagine finishing your 70-minute walk in 40 minutes — or the additional calories you'll burn by keeping up the pace for the full 70 minutes.

Your workout become more exciting: Turning up your intensity in short intervals can add variety to your exercise routine.

You can do without special equipment. You can simply modify your current routine.

Dancing

Aerobic dance workouts and exercises is extremely useful in helping to improve cardiovascular capacity by raising the overall use of oxygen in our body and ensuring that the heart works with full efficiency and capacity using less effort. This form of exercise not only provide health benefits but provide improved overall level of consciousness and alertness, decreased stress level, and improved cardiopulmonary health. It is highly recommended that this form of exercise be done at least 15 minutes daily and a minimum of three times a week to get full benefits of aerobic dance workouts and to achieve a better level of fitness.

In order to make it more exciting, you can use any of your favorite music like hip hop, jazz, or pop in your daily routine.

Aerobic dance can be so much fun and is easy to practice. Aerobic dance is very popular in many different countries. Some famous personalities like Jane Fonda and Sydney Rome contributed a great deal in making it very popular. After they discovered the fun and excitement in aerobic dance exercise and also its extraordinary effects on the human body decided to contribute by making it known worldwide.

A book called "aerobics" was first published in the United States of America in 1968. The author of the book "aerobics" was Dr. Kenneth H. Cooper, who was a physician of the United States Armed Forces in 1968. He outlined in his book that aerobics is a training program that he initially designed for members of the armed forces of his country which then spread and became popular in millions of people around the world. There are also some historical sources which attribute the term "aerobics" to Pasteur (France 1875).

Dr. Cooper's aerobic program included efforts in order to increase the endurance and performance of the user, thereby reducing percentage of risk to heart diseases like cardiovascular stroke and arteriosclerosis and also respiratory diseases. In the earlier chapters of the book "aerobics", Dr. Cooper has taught the virtues of aerobic exercise and the practice of physical exercise of low and medium intensity. The main objective of aerobics is the development of the cardiovascular system. He also defined in his book that aerobic training is a physical activity that can be done for prolonged period of time and is helpful in maintaining the balance between supply and consumption of oxygen if done in that manner. Oxygen is our body's need for energy production.

Walking

Walking is also one of the best and most valuable aerobic exercises

The benefit of walking is that it has less impact than running, and therefore less chances of injury. Anybody who is mobile can walk. But not everyone can run.

You don't need to pay any money to walk, and you don't require any equipment whatsoever. You only need a good pair of trainers.

Walking is as good as running

"Mile for mile walking burns almost as many calories as running does, as long as you walk fast."

This is true if you walk the same number miles as you run. It just means that if you walk, you have to do it longer in order to cover the same distance. Some study shows that duration of exercise is just as important as intensity.

Walking Reduces Stress

Studies have showed that women who walk (or are otherwise physically active) can have lower stress during their transition in menopause. This is from a study consisting of 360 women over the span of 9 years. Although physical symptoms of menopause such as hot flashes were no different.

Walking also reduces your risk of getting depression and decreases depression symptoms.

Aerobic Exercise Help Prevent Alzheimer

We know that aerobic exercise is good for the heart and the brain. In fact, aerobic exercise can help prevent Alzheimer's. Walking is aerobic exercise as long as one walks fast. The important points to note are: to walk briskly and to do it consistently and regularly.

A study in Hawaii involving 3000+ elderly men showed that regular walking is associated with decreased risk of dementia. The group who walked less than 0.35 mile per day had a 1.7-fold increase in risk of dementia than the group who walked more than 3 miles a day.

Part of the six-week Ultra Mind Solution, the prescription for the exercise portion is to "walk vigorously for thirty minutes every day.

Benefits of exercise in general:

Help prevents insulin resistance.

It increases neurotransmitters such as GABA, serotonin, and dopamine.

Reduces inflammation.

Increases neuroplasticity.

Increases neurogenesis (regeneration of brain cells)

Increases brain-derived neurotrophic factor (BDNF)

Aerobic exercise gets the lungs to breathe more deeply and the heart pumping. This improves circulation and improves blood flow to all parts of the body. All cells needs good circulation to get its oxygen and to eliminate waste.

With aerobic exercise your body releases endorphins which are sometimes called feel-good hormones because they give you a sense of well-being and are a natural pain killer. Therefore, it can help reduce anxiety and promote relaxation.

Aerobic exercise enhances the immune system so you can ward off the common cold or flu. It improves blood pressure and helps control sugar levels in your blood. It raises HDL (the good cholesterol) and decreases LDL (the bad cholesterol). It helps strengthens the heart and over time build endurance.

There have even been some studies that suggests that exercise (both aerobic and resistance training) helps decrease chronic inflammation as indicated by C-reactive protein markers.

Benefits of walking

Walking, like other exercise, can help you achieve a number of important health benefits as shown below:

Lower low-density lipoprotein (LDL) cholesterol (the "bad" cholesterol)

Raise high-density lipoprotein (HDL) cholesterol (the "good" cholesterol)

Lower your blood pressure

Reduce your risk of or manage type 2 diabetes

Manage your weight

Improve your mood

Stay strong and fit

All it takes to reap these benefits is a routine of vigorous walking. It doesn't get much simpler than that and you can forget the "no pain, no gain" talk. Research shows that regular, brisk walking can reduce the risk of heart attack by the same amount as more vigorous exercise, such as jogging.

A good walk cures most problems. Want to lose weight and get fit? Walk. Want to enjoy life but spend less? Walk. Want to cure stress and clear your head? Walk. Want to meditate and live in the moment? Walk. Having trouble with a life or work problem? Walk and your head gets clear."

Besides getting you fit, walking can clear your thoughts.

Cycling

Cycling is also one of the most beneficial aerobic exercises

Cycling leisurely for 30 minutes regularly several times in the week (about 3-4 times a week) ensures a better blood circulation in your entire body so the brain gets its fair share of nourishment and oxygen required for high mental activity.

Cycling involves the regular rhythmic movement of the legs which in turn increases the rate of heart functioning.

# CHAPTER 3

## Pillar 3:

Regular Mental Exercises

What happens in the brain during a mental exercise?

During a mental exercise, there are immediate changes in the blood flow causing an increase in density of all the important dendrites as well as a stimulation of the synapses and dendrites connections.

In this way, intellectual stimulation promotes brain growth and protects against cognitive decline in humans. Neurogenesis takes place during mental stimulation.

What is Neurogenesis?

Neurogenesis is the term used to describe the recently discovered capacity of the human brain to grow new neurons. Our brain is not physically fixed, it is constantly changing, losing some neurons, growing some neurons, making or deleting connections, and we can encourage such growth by mental exercises.

It is important to challenge your brain to learn new and novel tasks, especially processes that you've never done before. Examples include square-dancing, chess, tai chi, yoga, or sculpture. Working with modeling clay is an especially good way for children to grow new connections. It helps develop agility and hand-brain coordination, (like controlling the computer mouse with your opposite hand occasionally). Traveling is another good way to stimulate your brain.

INTENSITY AND REGULARITY OF MENTAL EXERCISES:

It is important to note that the efficiency of the brain could fluctuate based on two important factors, the intensity and regularity of an individual's mental activity.

The degree to which an individual tasks his brain is very important. The healthy growth of the brain with continuous multiplication of neurocells, increased dendrites connections is more pronounced when the brain is given a good measure of stimulation ( through mental exercises ) but what is more important is the regularity with which the brain is exercised.

Definitions

The intensity is the degree to which the brain is stimulated which includes the degree to which the brain is tasked or exercised.

The regularity of brain stimulation refers to involving the brain in a well spaced out program of mental exercises continuously throughout life. This does not have to be fixed as long as the individual by virtue of his occupation engages his mind in tasks that will keep the brain regularly stimulated such as regularly writing reports, checking and balancing accounts (for accountants and businessmen), attending board meetings (for top business executives) and so on.

Comparing the intensity with the regularity of mental exercise.

Let me explain why the regularity is more important than the intensity of the mental exercise. There is increased blood flow to the brain cells, growth and development of the brain cells only at the actual time the process of mental exercise and stimulation is taking place.

A long as the exercises remain regular and continuous, the brain cells are bound to remain alive, healthy with good rate of growth and development.

This is the secret to a healthy active brain that is fortified to battle with external invasion and diseases such as Alzheimer's.

The regularity of mental exercises goes a long way in determining a man's mental capacity. At periods when the mind is not engaged in tasks that will keep the brain cells stimulated, the rate of growth is reduced accordingly. If such periods are allowed to persist and are more prolonged than periods of brain stimulation, then there will be a gradual deterioration in mental performance irrespective of who is involved here.

Bearing this in mind, it is obvious that to a large extent, an individual's brain capacity and mental performance depends largely on him.

In developing a growing child's brain capacity, apart from feeding the child with the appropriate brain nourishments, a well planned and spaced out simple program of mental exercise has to be strictly adhered to.

Before I proceed to give you the various forms of mental exercises that exist, it is good to understand that any form of complex thinking in which the mind is adequately stretched to create workable ideas in order to solve an existing problem or create opportunity for improvement of one's life and that of other's is a very good form of mental exercise and is very useful for conditioning and trimming the brain.

Such exercises if consistent will go a long way in keeping the brain performing at peak level always.

As a rule, it is advisable to start with warm up exercises that will only take a few minutes to loosen your mental muscles and prepare it for more tedious tasks ahead.

Then as time goes on, you can gradually add more tedious and stretching exercises with increased time frame for completion. You try to increase the consistence and frequency of the exercises until they become part of your daily routine.

As with physical exercises, most of these exercises are a bit difficult at the onset but with regular practice, they become easier.

Don't shy away from the difficult exercises because the more tasking the exercise is, the more they stretch your mind and build your brain.

To make it very easy to understand, I am going to classify the mental exercises into the following categories:

(1) Visualization (Mental Rehearsal) and Creativity (Idea generation)

(2) Mental Calculations and Mind stretching games.

(3) Concentration and memory building exercises.

(4) Positive Thinking and idea generation.

(5) Exercises to train your power of logic.

(6) Reading.

(7) Neurobics

Regularly practicing some or all of these exercises help train and develop your brain power.

Mental Calculations and Mind Stretching Games:

Mental Calculations

Performing mental calculations using visual variations is a very good exercise for building your power of concentration as well as memory.

This exercise involves using your "mind's eye" to see figures on the blackboard. However small or large these numbers are, you visualize using your power of imagination to see the numbers as vividly as possible.

You now do addition, subtraction, multiplication or division with your focused mind and without the use of a calculator.

Always remember that, just like every other physical or mental exercises, it is always more difficult at the beginning but with consistent practice it becomes easier and even a second nature to you.

Let me give an example, you could start by working with much smaller numbers such as 1 X 2 = 2. Now you erase the

1 and visualize the 2 X 3 = 6. Now you erase the 2 and visualize the rest numbers.

This process is to continue until the figures are larger and more difficult to calculate. As time goes on, you will be spending several extra minutes at a time.

Just like every other exercises, the secret to success is repetition.

The more consistent and longer the time you spend on the exercise, the more effective and better this exercise strengthens your "mental muscles".

Just like all other exercises, it helps to reduce the effect of aging on your mental abilities as the brain cells enlarge and communicate better with such consistent stimulation irrespective of your age.

Problem Solving

Research on the physical results of thinking has shown that just using the brain actually increases the number of dendritic branches that interconnect brain cells. The more we think and stretch our minds to solve existing problems, the better our brains function – regardless of age. The renowned brain researcher Dr. Marian Diamond says, "The nervous system possesses not just a 'morning' of plasticity, but an 'afternoon' and an 'evening' as well."

Dr. Diamond found that whether we are young or old, we can continue to learn. The brain can change at any age. A dendrite grows much like a tree – from trunk to limbs to branches to twigs – in an array of ever finer complexity.

In fact, older brains may have an advantage. She discovered that more highly developed neurons respond even better to intellectual enrichment than less developed ones do. The greatest increase in dendritic length occurred in the outermost dendritic branches, as a reaction to new information.

As she poetically describes it: "We began with a nerve cell, which starts in the embryo as just a sort of sphere. It sends its first branch out to overcome ignorance. As it reaches out, it is gathering knowledge and it is becoming creative. Then we become a little more idealistic, generous, and altruistic; but it is our six-sided dendrites which give us wisdom."

 Mind Stretching Games:

Consider your brain a muscle, and find opportunities to flex it. Always engage in anything that stimulates or tasks the brain to think. Any time you feel like engaging in a recreational activity, it is advisable that you play games which require you to focus your mind and make better use of your intellect such as jigsaw puzzle and crossword puzzles. The more complicated the game is, the better. Three or four dimensional interlocking puzzles, board games such as checkers, chess, scrabble etc.

These games challenge your mind, compelling you to think and project yourself into the future, anticipating your opponent's next move in order to outsmart him.

So, anytime you feel like relaxing with a nice game, involve yourself with any of these above mentioned or any other mind stretching game that will eventually sharpen your overall intellect and make you smarter. Avoid games that depend on luck to win.

Here are some other examples of mind stretching games:

(a)  Word search puzzles.

(b)  Brain teasers (There are so many kinds of mind stretching brain   teasers to solve.)

(c)  Bridge games

(d)  Mind sharpening computer games

Keep your brain cells alive with mental exercises – Memory improvement exercises teach you to exercise your brain. These mental gymnastics strengthen nerve connections and activate little-used pathways in your brain to help keep your mind sharp.

Reading

Consider your brain a muscle, and find opportunities to flex it. Do a lot of reading says Dr. Amir Soas of Case Western Reserve University Medical School in Cleveland. Engage yourself with crossword puzzles. Play Scrabble. Challenging the brain early in life is crucial to building up more "cognitive reserve" to counter brain-damaging disease, according to Dr. David Bennett of Chicago's Rush University. And, reading-habits prior to age 18 are a key predictor of later cognitive function.

Start a new hobby or learn to speak a new  language. It is also advisable to watch less television, as this does not stretch the mind in anyway.

Form the habit of reading a lot. Read, read, and read. Reading and recollecting what you have read is a very good exercise for the brain. Never stop reading at any age. Research has shown that a lot of reading can improve your IQ irrespective of your age.

Mental Rehearsal (Visualization and Creativity):

Apart from fact that this is a very effective tool for enhancing creativity, it is also a strong tool for building a dependable memory.

From time to time, sit back and mentally rehearse and visualize whatever you want to recall easily.

For instance, when you are relaxed, you can mentally rehearse (several times) a new skill learned. However complex the new skill looks, try (initially with more effort) to picture in your "mind's eye" the step by step procedure in accomplishing the task. Do this for every new skill (e.g. computer skills) learnt.

Initially, when you start, it will take a lot more effort, but as time goes on, it becomes much easier with regular repetition, the visualized skill or action becomes registered in your long term memory and even becomes much easier to perform.

This mental visualization should be practiced when relaxed and comfortable. It does not matter what position you adopt as long as you are comfortable and can maintain that position for the whole practice period.

Note: Imagination is the key to improving your memory to a very dependable level. Imagination helps to strengthen your memory and using visual rehearsal helps to improve your imagination.

Always remember that initially, your imagination might be a little rusty but with consistent practice, you begin to visualize whatever you want to, more easily and even faster. This increases the speed with which you recall information.

Reminder: The golden rule to mastery is repetition. Practice makes perfect.

Developing your imagination is an invaluable exercise for meeting everyday challenges. Its gives you a total control over your memory and makes learning a lot easier.

Try developing your memory by using your "mind's eye" to see things regularly including names, numbers, places, past as well as forth coming events (such as forth coming work project and seminar presentation.), step by step procedure of a skill or technique etc.

As a mental practice, try to visualize vividly a forth coming event in order to figure out possible inadequacies or flames with a view to correcting it before the actual occurrence. Bring every minute detail into focus in your imagination, leaving no stone unturned.

Note: Visualization techniques can be very useful in storing information, learning, as well as in creativity. I encourage you to practice visualization regularly. It is one of the most useful personal assets that you could develop and it will improve your memory and creativity beyond expectation.

Use Visual Rehearsal to Master a Skill or Technique.

Whatever the skill is, whether in any sporting event such as golf, basketball, volleyball etc. computer skills, speech delivery, seminar presentation, debate etc. you can use visual rehearsal to master such a skill.

Procedure: When you are relaxed in a very comfortable position and have put away all forms of distractions from your mind, you can at will switch on your "mental cinema" and try as much as possible to visualize (putting every minute detail into focus) the step by step procedure of a particular skill or technique you wish to master. This should be done regularly to make it easier with each new effort.

Advantages: This regular practice, apart from helping you master such a skill desired, also helps you improve your memory drastically and also boosts your creative ability.

Remember: Like every new technique, initially mental picturing may seen difficult but becomes much easier with each new practice.

Use Visualization to create solutions to existing problems or create and modify ideas.

I will say it a hundred times and it still would not be enough; the value of visualization in building concentration, memory and creativity can never be overemphasized.

Use all your imaginative power to visualize or picture all the creative ways you can use to solve a problem or to work on an idea. As usual, bring every minute detail in to visual focus.

Visualization stages:

Creative Stage:

At this first stage, don't even consider whether the idea is feasible or whether it makes sense. Just allow the ideas flow in to full view, making use of the creative picture that comes to mind.

Use the creative language "What if" to picture or visualize several new ideas that could possibly be a solution to a problem, without criticizing or evaluating any forth coming visual image.

You can note all your ideas down in writing so that you do not loose useful ideas.

Analytical Stage;

This is the stage for criticism of ideas. The second stage is to visualize all practical considerations that will help the idea make sense and be achievable such as financial and human resources available, time factor etc.

Try as much as possible to be realistic and criticize every aspect of the idea, while staying constructive.

Write down the outcome of all your analysis.

Go through the creative and analytical stages over and over again until very practical, workable solution to every aspect of the problem is covered and taken care of.

By this process, you will find out that important weakness are being addressed and solved one by one.

Benefits of this exercise:

This exercise has the following benefits:

(1) Improve your concentration and memory tremendously.

(2) Help boost creativity drastically.

(3) Help strengthen your mental muscles and consequently your thinking ability.

(4) Help solve problems

(5) Help you create opportunities.


Developing Memory

Developing kinetic Memory:

One of the best ways to learn is by doing or taking action, even when you make mistakes, correct them and move on. Without making mistakes, you cannot learn or make progress.

Most times, when an individual conditions himself to depend on himself to perform most tasks (both personal and business), he usually becomes far more efficient in carrying out those functions than individuals who actually depend on others to carry out such tasks.

In the medical field, survey has shown that surgeons who are exposed to carrying out several surgeries in a week virtually become better experienced and more dependable to carry out sensitive and difficult surgery where utmost care is required.


Neurobics

This is a unique system of brain exercises using your five physical senses and your emotional sense in unexpected ways that encourage you to shake up your everyday routines. They are designed to help your brain manufacture its own nutrients that strengthen, preserve, and grow brain cells.

It was created by Lawrence C. Katz, Ph.D., a professor of neurobiology at Duke University Medical Center. Neurotics can be done anywhere, anytime, in offbeat, fun and easy ways. Nevertheless, these exercises can activate underused nerve pathways and connections, helping you achieve a fit and flexible mind.

# CHAPTER 4

## Pillar 4

Specific Lifestyle Habits

It is not enough to take the right brain nutrients, the kind of lifestyle an individual leads also goes a long way in affecting his mental efficiency.

For optimal mental performance you have to create room for or include in your daily routine a regular aerobic exercises or workout (At least thrice in a week).

You have to be consistently involved in social activities so as to offset brain laziness. Looking in this direction, it is also advisable to do a lot of reading, and be involved in one kind of recreational activity that requires problem solving like playing board games such as chess, checkers, etc.

Learn a new language or a new skill. Plan activities with friends and relatives and hang around positive people. Avoid hanging around negative people. Thinking positively stimulates the brain and brightens your day.

Research has shown that consistent challenge and activity can preserve a sound mind.

So the secret of engaging in planned recreational activities and socializing with others is that by constantly stimulating the brain and stretching the mind to create ideas (opportunities), solving problems of all sorts for others and engaging in intellectually stimulating discussions always help sharpen the intellect, keeping it young and active for a long time.

On the other hand, isolation can slow thinking and remembering. Believe me, when you stop using your mind, you start losing it and it begins to deteriorate with age faster.

Apart from socializing, it is of immense value to incorporate into your daily or weekly program a short period for creative mental exercises.

Its long term effect in strengthening the mental muscles is pronounced like the ones described in the previous chapter.


Specific Lifestyle Factors That Affect Mental Performance

Stress and Stress Management

There are various forms of stressor:  physical, mental or emotional.

Examples of Physical stressors are exposure to extremes of heat or cold involvement in car accident exposure to radiation, reaction to any serious illness, marathon running, and heavy lifting.

Examples of mental stressors include preparing for and taking an arduous exam or having to take a very difficult problem where the answer is not forth coming.

Examples of severe emotional stressors are death of a beloved one, deep seated hatred, and loss of a much valued job, anxiety and fear.

Effect of Stress on the Brain Cells: Under stress conditions, most of the glucose is diverted from the brain to other vital organs and muscle systems in response to the emergency there by depriving the brain of its rightful supply of oxygen and nutrients.


A brain area which plays a significant role in memory and mood control, the hippocampus, becomes seriously deprived of glucose. As a result of this, the cells in the by hippocampus become injured.

Sustained stress is damaging because prolonged glucose deprivation can bring about brain cell starvation and in extreme cases, brain cell death.

How to cope with stress:

It is not actually the stressor that undermines us but our attitude towards the stressor. Our response to stress is far more important than the stress itself.

Research has shown that those who stay healthy under stress had a different way of dealing with it.

For those who have developed to a high resistance to stress, it does not have much effect on their brain but those who have not developed a high tolerance to stress respond poorly to problems such that high levels of stress can do direct damage to their brain.

1)  Identifying and Uprooting the Stress

The first step in dealing with stress is to identify the stressor. Then the next step is to take remedial action.

 In other words, to effectively manage stress, it is advisable to first determine the causes of the stress, then deal with the basics, the underlying problems.

By getting rid of the underlying problems and getting rid of the causes of the stress, you are bound to be relieved from the stress.

(2) Relaxation and breathing Exercises

This is usually very beneficial when you are having a lot of anxious thoughts and when you are trying to quiet your mind.

Breathing exercise though appears very simple, is very effective in helping you relax completely. Now this relaxation technique involves your sitting upright and taking slow deep breathes.

Step 1

On sitting upright, you start by exhaling as much as possible in order to empty your lungs completely to enable you fill up your lungs with fresh oxygen.

Step 2

Then you inhale slowly but deeply and hold it for a count of eight. You now exhale completely once again. You repeat the entire process for up to ten times.

This simple breathing exercise in addition to helping you relax, also improves the amount of oxygen that gets to the brain and resultantly promotes mental efficiency drastically.

Note: This exercise is highly recommended before undergoing any form of mental exercise and before giving a public speech.

Useful under stressful situations because during such conditions, most people become shallow breathers.

Research also showed that when individuals are exposed to a subnormal level of oxygen in their environment and therefore subnormal level of oxygen in their system, they have difficulty in concentrating and their perception time become much slower, they suffer headaches, dizziness anxiety, depression reduced productivity and difficulty in remembering.

Sleep and mental activity

It is very important to note that adequate sleep is inevitable in maximizing one's mental efficiency.

Research shows that a minimum of between seven to eight hours sleep at night is very necessary to ensure optimal brain performance.

Without adequate sleep, the level of vital nutrients such as zinc and magnesium fall and vitamin C is used up at faster rate than normal. Resultantly, the level of one's thinking ability does not reach optimal level.

Considering this, it is advisable that when an individual only gets a few hours sleep at night (for some reason beyond his control) he should find time during the day (such as in afternoon) to make up for the lost sleep so as to optimize his mental efficiency.

Getting Adequate Sleep:

Knowing that getting adequate sleep is necessary to maximize your mental efficiency, every step must be taken to improve your sleep life and to cure insomnia (the inability to sleep).

If you are having problems getting enough sleep or staying asleep, there are appropriate steps to take to revert this but it is not advisable to use any form of medications (drugs) to induce sleep.

Reasons:

(1) Laxatives, tranquilizers, sedatives impair memory and affect other aspects of mental function.

(2) Some drugs which contain anti-histamine such as some meant for allergy and cold can induce drowsiness and affect one's ability to recall.

(3) Some cardiovascular drugs used to control high blood pressure (Such as propanolol) can also cause depression and memory weakness.

(4) Two or more drugs when taken together can interact with each other to affect one's mental efficiency.

Safer ways to ensure a sound sleep:

Using Calcium and Magnesium minerals

Calcium and magnesium minerals work together to relax the nerves and muscles thereby ensuring a sound sleep.

 A supplement of 600mg of Calcium and 400mg of Magnesium at bedtime will help induce a sound sleep

Also it is advisable to improve daily intake of calcium by including the following in your diet, nuts, seafood, green vegetables, and milk.

 To improve your intake of magnesium, it is advisable you include the following in your daily diet, green vegetables, seeds nuts, wholegrain and seafood.

1)  By regulating your blood–sugar level

Normal blood sugar level is important for optimal mental efficiency. Keeping your blood sugar levels within normal range during the day prepares you for the correct patterns  at night and gives you a better chance of a good night's sleep.

How can you regulate your blood sugar level?

By eating regular small meals throughout the day instead of settling down to two or three large meals.

Also, it is advisable that such meals include protein rich food such as fish, eggs or lean meat.

It is also advisable to avoid refined foods, coffee (a stimulant) sugary foods, and drinks.

2)  Making use of vitamin B6 & Tryptophan

Adequate amounts of vitamin B6 and tryptophan can also help you easily have a sound sleep at night. .

Foods that are particularly high in tryptophan are chicken, cheese, tuna, tofu, eggs, nuts, seeds, and milk.

So drinking a glass of milk at bedtime can also help naturally induce sleep.

Conclusion:

Your habits and lifestyle can go a long way in promoting your brain development.

Socializing

Research has shown that consistent challenge and activity can preserve a sound mind irrespective of age.

Note;

By engaging in planned recreational activities and socializing with others, there is a constant unconscious stimulation of your brain and also by stretching your mind to create ideas/ opportunities, to solve problems of all sorts for others and engaging in intellectually stimulating discussions, you sharpen your intellect, keeping it young and active for a long time.

On the other hand, when you isolate yourself for a prolonged period of time, you gradually, unconsciously slow your thinking and remembering. Also when you stop using your mind, you start to lose it and it begins to deteriorate with age faster.

Physical activity

For optimum mental performance you have to create room for or include in your daily routine or schedule regular aerobic exercises or workout (At least thrice in a week).

Create time out of your busy schedule to take long 20 to 30minutes walk on daily basis or at least several times in the week, as this will go a long way to improve your blood circulation and resultantly your mental efficiency.

Stress Management

It is not advisable to allow stress go uncontrolled for too long as prolonged uncontrolled stress is damaging to the brain for the fact that prolonged glucose deprivation can bring about brain cell starvation and in extreme cases, brain cell death.

Getting Adequate Sleep:

Knowing that getting adequate sleep is necessary to maximize your mental efficiency every step must be taken to improve your sleep life and to cure insomnia (the inability to sleep).

It is advisable for you to get at least 7 to 8hours night sleep. Where for some reason this is not possible, it is important that you make up for it with a sound afternoon sleep.

# CHAPTER 5

## Pillar 5:

Heavy Metals And Toxins That Destroy Brain Cells

Let's examine alcohol & mental Efficiency

What is the effect of alcohol on the brain cells?

Even a very small quantity such as an once of alcohol can cause spasm of arterioles (branches of arteries slightly larger than capillaries) and cuts off oxygen, a condition called hypoxia.

This reduced oxygen in brain and body first produces fuzzy mindedness, lack of concentration, weakness in the mental capabilities.

When more alcohol is consumed, more spasms of brain arteries occur resulting in impaired vision poor muscle co-ordination and unsteadiness.

Arteriole constriction at this point can be extreme enough to cut off completely oxygen carrying blood and resultantly damage brain cells or networks of them (either temporally or permanently).

When the damage caused in the brain cell covers is large enough area it could result in stroke.

Bearing all these in mind, it is advisable to avoid alcohol completely in order to maximize your mental powers.

Tobacco and Mental Health

Effect of smoking on the brain: How does smoking sabotage the mind?

Although nicotine is a brain stimulant just like caffeine, it depresses thyroid gland function, so in the long run smoking certainly deteriorates thinking & remembering. It does so by constricting the blood vessels. Research shows that it can even narrow blood vessels for as much as 40 minutes throughout the brain and body.

Poor blood circulation to the brain cells also reduces the amount of oxygen and nutrients being carried by red blood cells to them.  The consequence of this is reduced mental efficiency such as deterioration in memory and thinking capabilities.

Secondly, the tobacco smoke also gives off carbon monoxide which displaces some oxygen in the red blood capsules, causing an even greater oxygen deficit. Just like before, the result is weakness in mental function.

Nutrients that protect from tobacco smoking:

(1) Vitamin A

Taking large daily supplements such as 5,000 to 10,000 International units of vitamin A offers some protection to vulnerable mucus membranes of the throat and lungs.

So it is advisable to eat foods and supplements that are rich in vitamin A such as cod liver oil, carrots, red peppers, egg yolk, white fish, water melon, mackerel, yams and beef liver.

(2) Antioxidants

Other very good protective nutrients are anti-oxidants such as vitamin E and C. Taking 800 1.U.s of vitamin E (D-alpha tocopherol) is also very useful against tobacco smoking.

Also vitamin C protects against a wide range of pollutants in tobacco smoke. Vitamin C also helps to restore vitamin E (to free radical fighting) when it is depleted.

(3)Zinc

A daily intake of 15mg to 30mg zinc helps to keep the immune system strong against pollutants from smoking.

Some heavy metals that destroy brain cells and deteriorate mental performance

This section deals with heavy metals, how they find their way into our system, cause several mental setbacks, and finally how they can be got rid of from our system.

Copper

Copper which is classified as an essential mineral can also be toxic.

Sources

(1) Excess Copper in our system may result from drinking water passing through copper pipes, copper pots and pans, the contraceptive pills.

(2)It may be as a result of deficiency in zinc, vitamin B3, Vitamin C.

Consequence of excess Copper.

Copper excess can cause:

1) Extreme fear, paranoia and hallucinations.

2) Poor attention Span.

3) Hyperactivity.

4) Aggressive behavior.

Prevention

To avoid taking in excess copper into your system, it is advisable to drink filtered or bottled water.

Mercury

This is very toxic indeed and on reaching the brain cells, it disturbs brain function and makes an individual crazy. It also causes headaches and memory loss.

 Sources

1) Small amounts enter our body through contaminated food.

2) From dental tooth fillings.

3) Eating fish caught from mercury polluted waters.

Aluminum

When this metal gets into the brain, it results in memory disorder diseases such as Alzheimer's.

Sources:

1) Toothpaste tubs

2) Aluminum foil

3) Aluminum pots and pans

4) Aluminum pipes contamination water flow

5) Antacids,

6) Toothpaste tubes

7) Food packaging with aluminum materials

Lead

Lead toxicity can result in the following in children:

1) Aggressive outbursts

2) Sinus conditions

3) Inability to concentrate

4) Disturbed sleep patterns

5) Can create irreversible brain damage.

Lead toxicity can cause the following in adults:

1) Lack of mental energy

2) Insomnia and restlessness

3) Confusion, irritability

4) Anxiety

5) Delusions

6) Depression

7) Neurological problems

8) Headaches and convulsions

Cadmium

This also disturbs mental performance and cause increased aggression.

Sources:

1) The most common source is cigarettes.

2) Car exhaust fumes.

3) Small amounts can enter our system through food.


Detoxifying the brain of heavy metals:


(1)Vitamin C

Once lead has entered into the brain where it causes most damage, it is very difficult to remove.

Vitamin–C is very effective in removing lead and cadmium from the brain since it can readily cross the blood brain barrier. So it attaches to most heavy metals in the blood stream and brings them out of the system.


(2) Zinc (Usually as zinc gluconate)

Zinc is another substance that protects against heavy metals such as lead by preventing it's absorption in the gut (Stomach). Zinc also lowers brain levels of cadmium. So zinc supplements (as zinc gluconate) are highly beneficial to most people.

## (3) Calcium

Calcium is very effective in keeping the levels of aluminum, lead and cadmium down. Maintaining a good level of calcium in the body also prevents the rapid rise of toxic heavy metals in the system.

## Control your Alcohol consumption

Even a very small quantity such as an once of alcohol can cause spasms of arterioles (branches of arteries slightly larger than capillaries) and cuts off oxygen, a condition called hypoxia.

This reduced oxygen in body and brain first produces fuzzy mindedness, lack of concentration, weakness in the mental capabilities.

Bearing all these in mind, it is advisable to avoid alcohol completely in order to maximize your mental powers.

## Control your tobacco smoking

Although nicotine is a brain stimulant just like caffeine, it depresses thyroid gland function, so in the long run smoking certainly deteriorates thinking & remembering. I strongly advise that you even try as much as possible to avoid passive smoking i.e. hanging around people smoking.

Watch the water you drink

Most of the heavy metals which are toxic and gradually destroy the brain cells can be found in untreated water. So it is advisable to be more cautious about the water you drink.

To avoid taking in excess Copper, Aluminum, Mercury, Lead and some other heavy metals into your system, it is advisable to drink filtered or bottled water.

Watch the kind of cooking pots and pans you use

Copper pots and pans, Aluminum pots and pans slowly release these harmful metals into the food being prepared with them and finally they find their way into the brain where they cause severe harm such as Alzheimer's disease (a memory disorder disease) as in the case of aluminum.

Bearing all these in mind, it is very necessary to cultivate the habits and lifestyle that will go a long way in maximizing your brain power.

# Acknowledgments

First and foremost, I'd like to say a big thanks to the

Almighty God who made it possible for me to carry out my

research and to give my own fair contribution to mental
health care.


Secondly, to my lovely and caring wife for her support,
understanding and encouragement when the project was
taking a great deal of my time, even when I had to get back
home very late quite so often.

88

# About the Author

Dr. Peter C. Omoghene, who graduated from the University of Benin in 1998, is an experienced Optometrist, Low Vision Specialist (B.Sc, OD) and a Mental health researcher (MHR) with many years of ground breaking discoveries in mental healthcare that has helped millions of people avoid age related mental decline and stay mentally fit throughout their lives.

His main goal in mental health has always been to teach interested individuals how to use the five pillars such as nutrition, aerobic exercise, lifestyle, mental exercise and knowledge about toxic substances to stay mentally fit throughout their lives.

Even as new technology evolves in a dynamic world like ours, he strives to stay informed and give updates on the latest strategies that may improve the mental health and well being of all those who read his books.

# Other books written by author:

## 99% Maximize Your Vision

### Dr. Peter C. O.

99% Maximize Your Vision reveals the four pillars that help to maximize your vision. Multiple nutrients that your eyes need to transform light into electrical signals, thereby boosting your vision.

Free radicals and toxins that harm your eyes, deteriorate your vision and cause silent eye blinding diseases. The recommended daily nutrients you need to protect your eyes from such oxidative damage.

Daily exercises you need to strengthen your ocular muscles and improve your vision.

All the information you need to protect your eyes from silent eye blinding diseases has been simplified by a low vision specialist.

www.ingramcontent.com/pod-product-compliance
Lightning Source LLC
Chambersburg PA
CBHW070744250726
48662CB00004B/1633